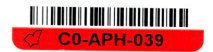

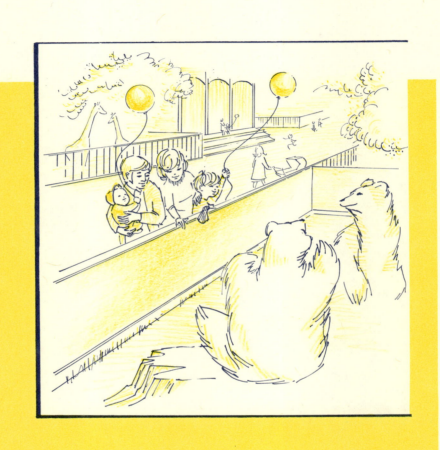

BILLY AND OUR NEW BABY

by

Helene S. Arnstein

Behavioral Publications
New York

Library of Congress Cataloging in Publication Data

Arnstein, Helene S
   Billy and our new baby.

   SUMMARY: Feeling jealous of his new baby brother,
Billy wants to behave like a baby but realizes that
it's more fun to be a big boy.
   [1. Brothers and sisters—Fiction]
I. Smyth, M. Jane, illus. II. Title.
PZ7.A739Bi   [E]   73-7951
ISBN 0-87705-093-7

Library of Congress Catalog Number 73-7951
Standard Book Number 87705-093-7
Copyright © 1973 by Behavioral Publications

BEHAVIORAL PUBLICATIONS
2852 Broadway—Morningside Heights,
New York, New York 10025

Printed in the United States of America
This printing   10 9 8 7 6 5 4 3 2 1

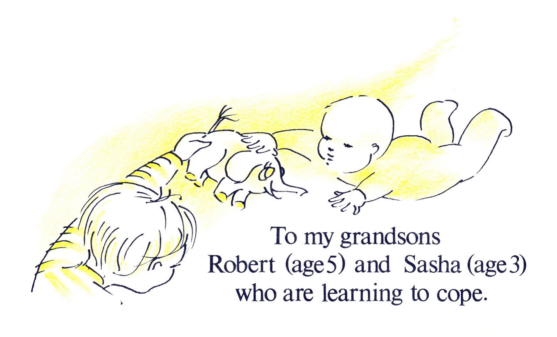

To my grandsons
Robert (age 5) and Sasha (age 3)
who are learning to cope.

Daddy brought Mommy home from the hospital and
   said,
"Billy, here is Our New Baby."
Billy rushed over and handed Baby one of his best toy
   cars.
But Baby was too little to hold the car.
Billy felt disappointed and sad.
You see, he'd been told he would have a baby to play
   with.

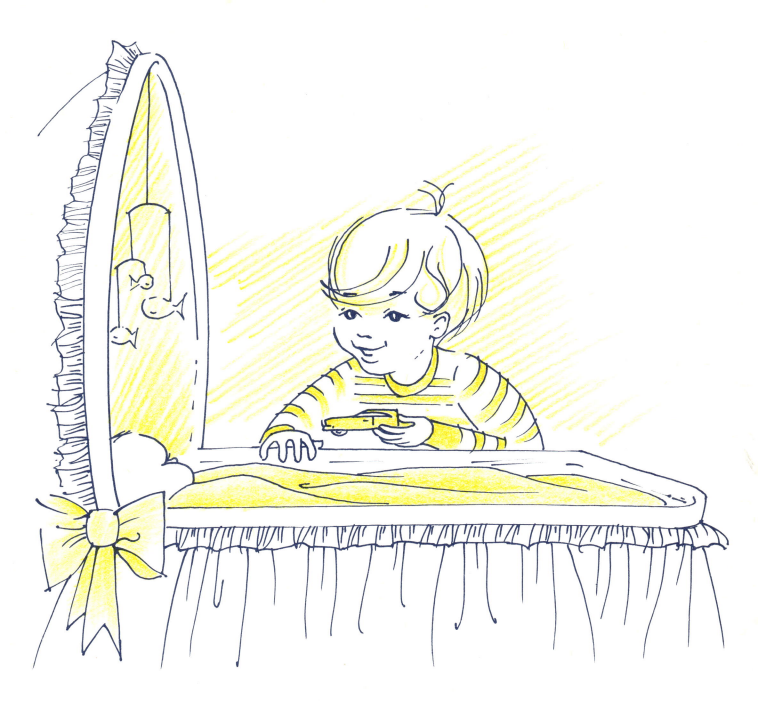

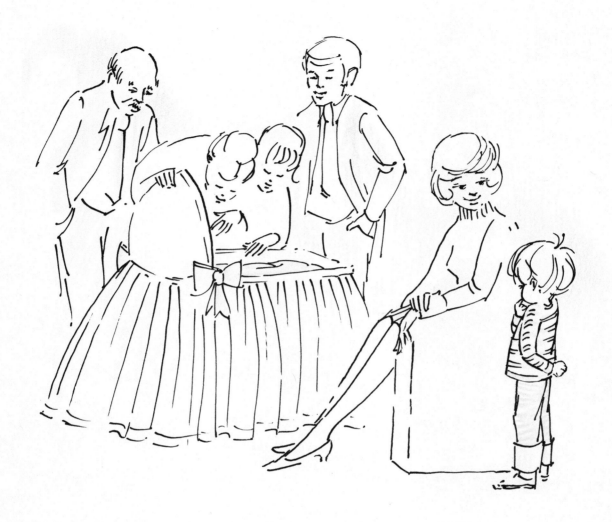

Billy felt angry because everyone fussed over that tiny
    little baby.
And that baby couldn't do anything but eat and sleep
    and cry!

"Watch *me*! Watch me!" shouted Billy.
And he threw his ball high into the air.

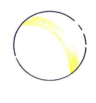

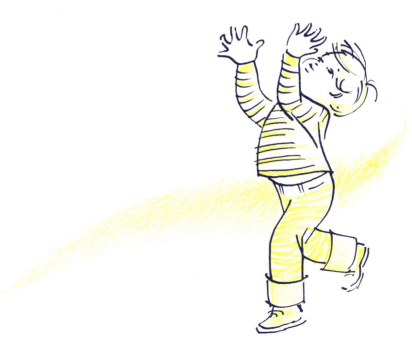

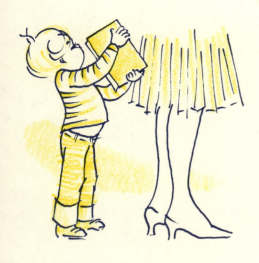

Billy often asked Mommy to play with him or read him
  a story.
And she would say,

"I can't read to you or play with you now, darling,
I am busy with Our New Baby."

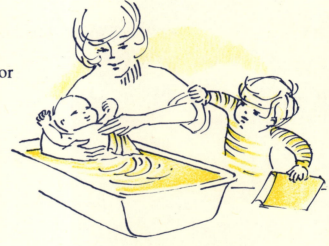

Mommy was always feeding or bathing Baby or
  changing Baby's diapers.
Billy didn't like that.

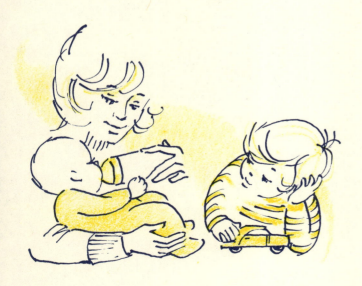

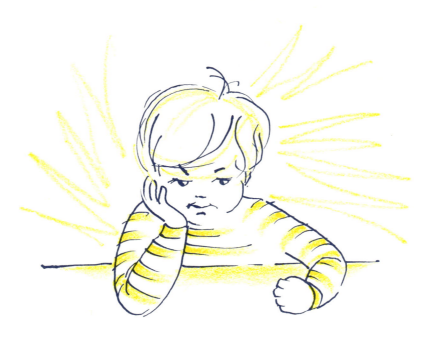

Billy felt angry at Mommy.
"Maybe Mommy loves the baby more than she loves
    me," thought Billy.

Billy had an idea.
Things would be all right again if Baby would go away!

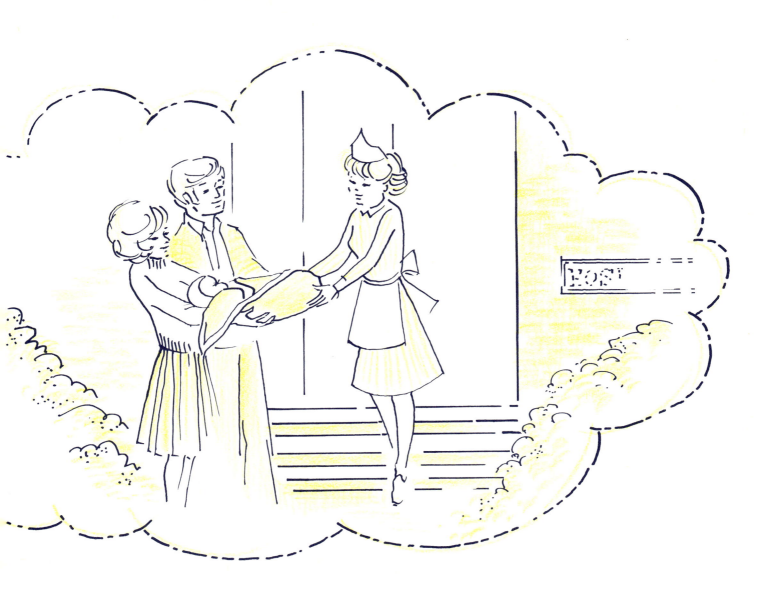

Maybe Mommy and Daddy could bring him back to the
  hospital where he was born.
So he ran over to Mommy and said happily, ''Let's take
  Baby back to the hospital!''

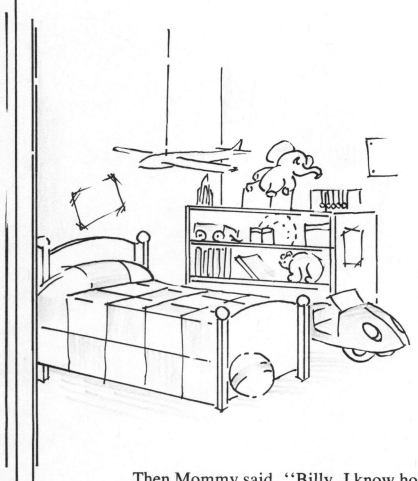

Then Mommy said, "Billy, I know how you feel.

Other little boys and girls who have a new baby in the
family feel the way you feel sometimes.

But Our New Baby belongs in our family just as you
do.

He belongs in our home.

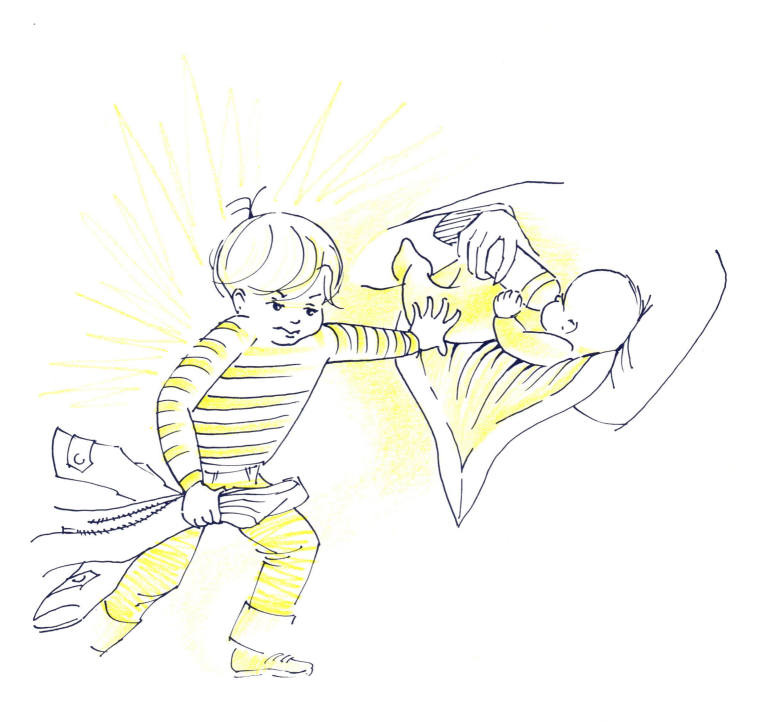

But Mommy gently stopped him.

She said, "Billy, I know how you feel.

You are angry because I have no time for you just now.

But I can't let you hurt Our New Baby.

And I wouldn't let anyone hurt *you*!"

Billy went over to his toys and made one of his cars roll
     real hard on the floor.

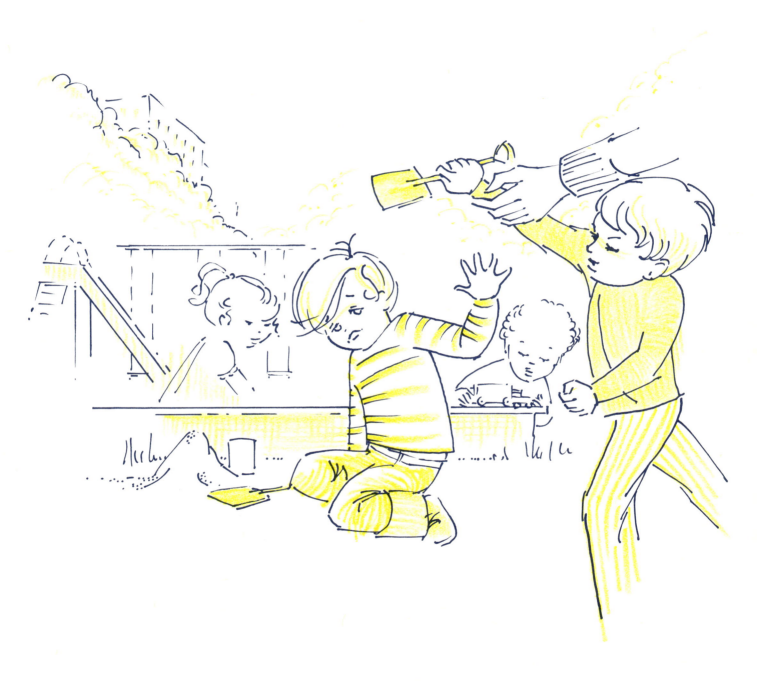

Soon Mommy said, "Now I'm ready. Come onto my
    lap for our own time together.
Bring me your favorite book and I'll read it to you
    before we go out.
Remember that I love you in a very special way. You're
    my special big boy, Billy."

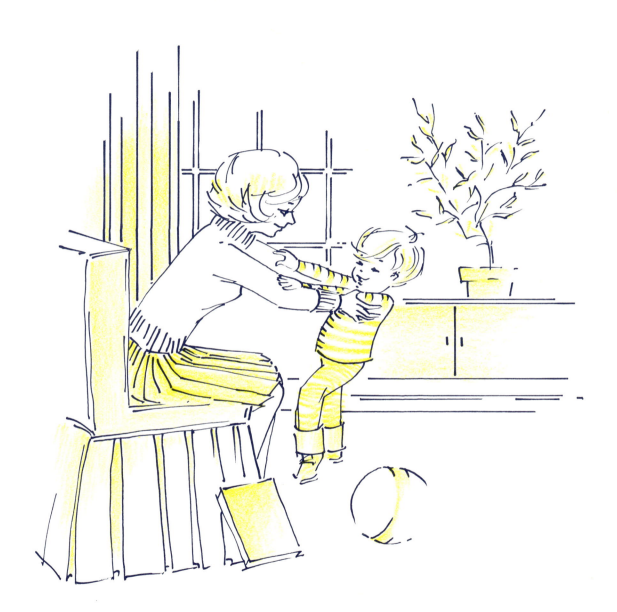

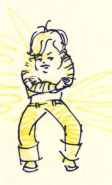

Billy said he didn't want to be a Special Big Boy.
"I want to be a baby," Billy said.
And do you know what Billy did?
He acted just like he did when he was a baby.

Billy began to crawl and creep again.

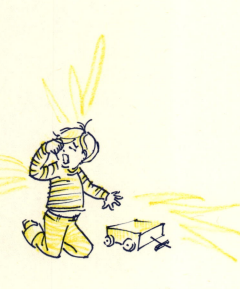

He cried a lot too.

Then suddenly Billy decided he wanted a bottle on Mommy's lap just like Baby.

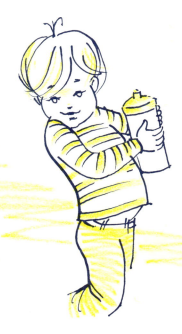

And Mommy said, ''Sure, Billy. Play like a baby if you
  wish.
Sure you can have a bottle on my lap.

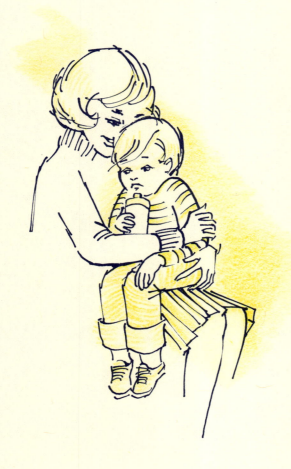

But you can get more out of a cup when you're hungry
    and thirsty.''
And Mommy was right.
It was hard to get milk out of the nipple.
And it didn't taste as good as milk from a cup.

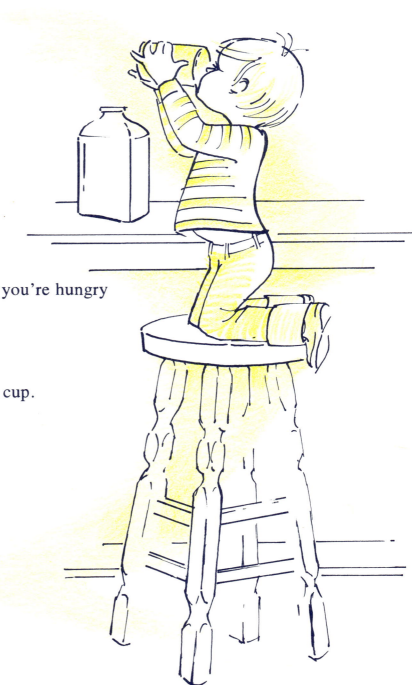

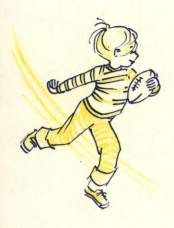

"You know, Billy," Mommy said, smiling, "*You* can run and jump.

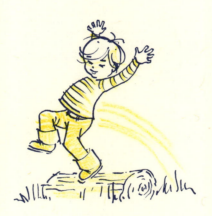

You can climb up the slide and slide down it.

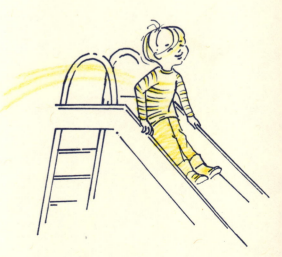

You can swing on a swing.

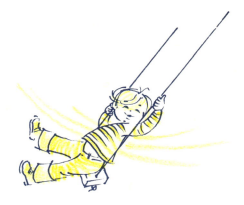

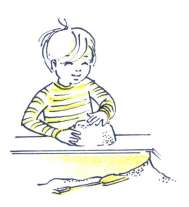

You can even make sand pies and ride in your new big
red car.

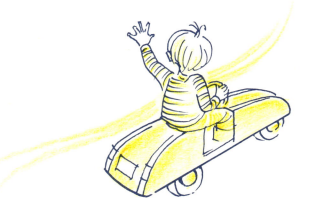

Baby can't do these things.
You can be a baby if you want to.
But it's more fun to be a big boy."

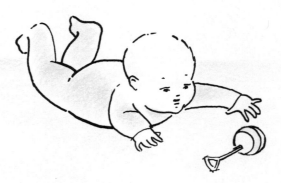

Billy laughed then and said,
"Yes! Baby can only eat and sleep and cry.

Billy can run and jump and do a lot of things."
I'm a *big boy*! Baby is only a *baby*!"

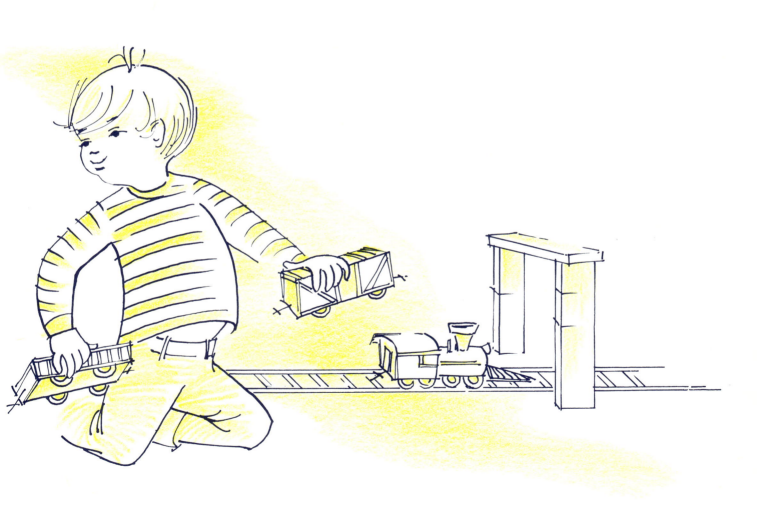

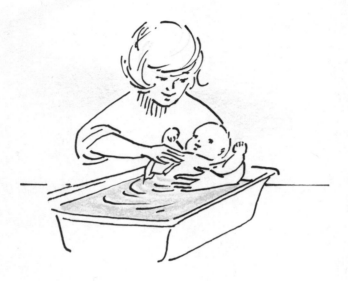

That evening Mommy was giving Baby a bath as usual.
Billy decided to help her and ran to Mommy with
Baby's clean diaper.

Mommy was happy and she smiled and said,
"Thank you, thank you, Billy. You can really be a big
   help!"
Billy felt proud that he could help.

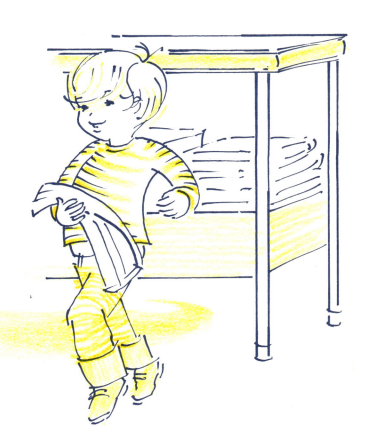

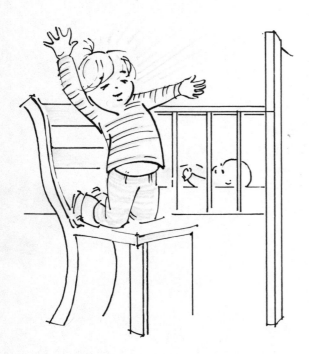

Then one day Billy climbed onto a chair near Baby's
    crib.
Billy made funny faces and waved to the baby.
Then he called to Mommy and Daddy all excited.
"Mommy, Daddy, Our New Baby smiled at me!"
Maybe soon the baby would be big enough to play with
    him!
"And maybe," thought Billy, "the baby can come
    along to the zoo with Mommy, Daddy and me.
    Baby can see all the animals too."

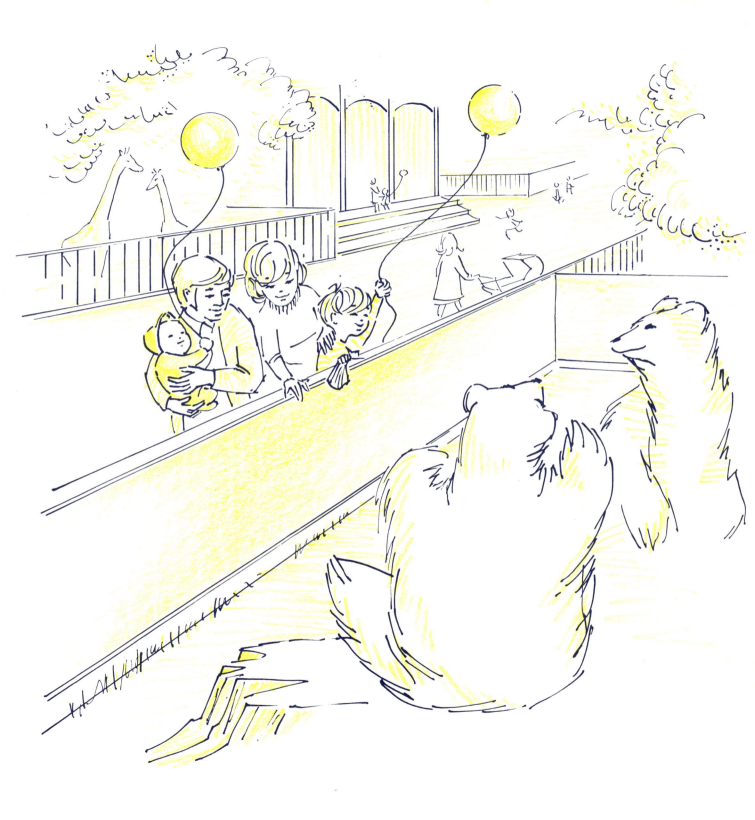

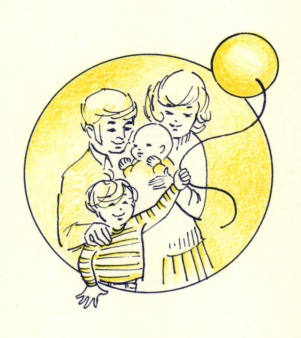

But Billy still got mad at the new baby at times.

Sometimes he got mad for good reasons and sometimes just because the baby made him angry.

Billy knew that other little children also felt this way sometimes when they had a new baby in the family.

Yet there were those other times when Billy loved the baby and had fun with him.

Billy was really beginning to feel now that Our New Baby belonged to him too.

Of course! Our New Baby was part of Our Family.

GUIDE FOR PARENTS AND THOSE
WHO WORK WITH CHILDREN

This book is aimed at helping the pre-schooler make his adjustment to a new baby in the family.

Up to now this very young "older" child has been the star performer on stage. Suddenly he finds that he must share the stage and spotlight with a new starlet. Quite an undertaking and adjustment for one so young and inexperienced! The very young child is often caught up in conflicting and painful feelings he doesn't understand and sometimes can't even express in words. Therefore he may express his feelings in behavior that may be hard for a parent to understand, or hard for parents to take. (The overly "good" child's needs also should not be underestimated).

Jealousy and anger are perfectly normal emotions and quite appropriate at this time. These emotions cannot be suppressed altogether, but the child can be helped in learning how to cope with and better handle his feelings. He may gradually become aware of the fact that while it is all right to *feel* angry he may not act in any way that is harmful to the younger child or destructive to others. And down deep he wants to know he is being protected from his own angry impulses.

When the older child is helped to see that he is not the only child who feels the way he does, and that he is not "bad" because he has such feelings, these negative and uncomfortable feelings—including the inevitable guilt —may diminish, giving room for the appearance and growth of positive feelings of love and protectiveness for the newcomer.

Naturally, each child is different. There are some, who although toilet-trained, decide to forget it for a while. Or maybe they want to be helped in getting dressed even though a short while ago they were proud of being able to open and close zippers and buttons. All of this sudden helplessness is really a ploy for reassurance of continuing love, affection and attention. Some extra time with mother and father may help the older child see that the newcomer has not replaced him in their love. Usually these regressive behaviors are short-lived; they vanish in good time and the older child moves on towards further strides in his development and maturing.

Should a mother be breast-feeding her baby instead of bottle-feeding and find herself in the awkward position of being asked for the breast, some authorities suggest she might gently point out to her older child that it is only very little babies who nurse at the breast, but if he (or she) would like it Mother might hold him close in the same way as the baby and let him try a bottle—if he thinks he really wants this. His demand is apt to imply, "Can you love me as much as you love this little baby and will I get more love and attention if I become a baby again?" Appropriate answers to some of the firstborn's unspoken (or spoken) questions may be found in the text of this book.

Before, during and after the time of the birth of a new baby a child may become curious about a number of things. He may want to know how the baby was born, and, if the baby is of the opposite sex, why are the genitals different, etc. These questions cannot be dealt with here but there are many books available that can help parents and teachers find a way in which to respond to such questions.